ANA MARIA SANTOS

Sleeping for Two

A Guide to a Healthy Sleep Routine During Pregnancy

This book is dedicated to all pregnant women, who embark on a unique and transformative journey. To women who face the physical and emotional changes of pregnancy with courage and determination. To all mothers, who have the power to create life and nurture unconditional love. And to the loving and supportive companions, who are at the side of pregnant women, supporting them every step of the way.

May this book be a compassionate and inspiring guide, offering useful and practical information for a restful sleep routine during pregnancy. May it bring comfort, knowledge and confidence, helping to create an environment conducive to restorative rest.

To all future mothers, I wish you a peaceful pregnancy, full of moments of joy and connection. May you find comfort and balance during your sleep, so that you can experience a healthy and rewarding pregnancy experience.

With love,

Ana Maria Santos

summary

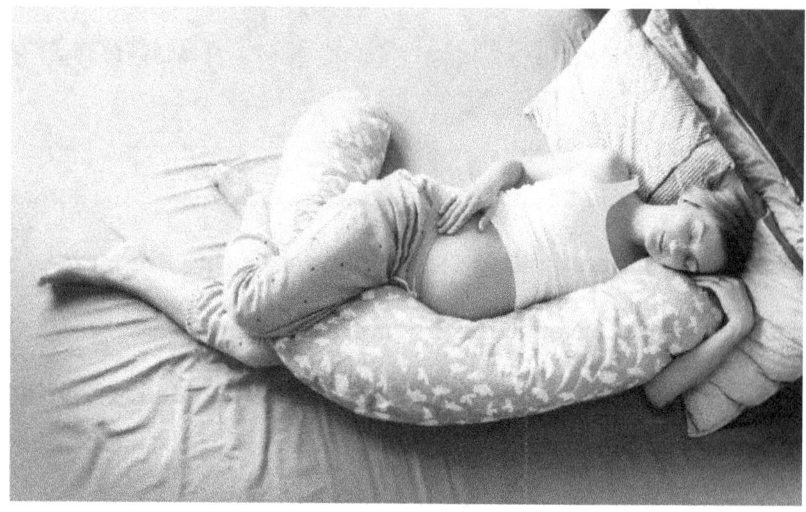

Introduction

Congratulations on your pregnancy and on your search for information that will contribute to your well-being and that of your baby. During this special time in your life, sleep plays a crucial role in your physical, mental and emotional health.

Pregnancy brings with it a series of physical, hormonal and emotional changes that can affect sleep patterns. It is common to experience challenges such as difficulty finding a comfortable position, increased urinary frequency, physical discomfort and even nighttime worries and anxieties.

These changes can interfere with the quality and quantity of sleep, resulting in restless nights and daytime tiredness.

Understanding and addressing these challenges is essential to ensuring a healthy sleep routine during pregnancy. This book is designed to provide comprehensive, practical information on how to improve the quality of your sleep and promote a restful, revitalizing sleep routine for you and your baby.

Throughout this book, we'll explore the factors that affect sleep during pregnancy, the specific sleep needs of pregnant women, common challenges faced during this time, and effective strategies for improving sleep quality. We'll also discuss the impact of sleep on your maternal health and fetal development, as well as additional care, special considerations, and preparation for your baby's arrival.

Remember that each pregnancy is unique, and the strategies that work for one pregnant woman may not be the same for another. It is important to listen to your body, seek appropriate professional support and adapt recommendations to your individual needs.

This book is an informative and practical guide to help you understand, address, and overcome sleep challenges during pregnancy. We hope that the information provided here will help you to establish a healthy sleep routine, enjoy peaceful nights and wake up revitalized and ready to make the most of this unique phase of your life.

Get ready to embark on a journey of discovery and learning about sleep during pregnancy. Let's explore together the strategies and care needed to ensure a healthy sleep routine for you and your baby

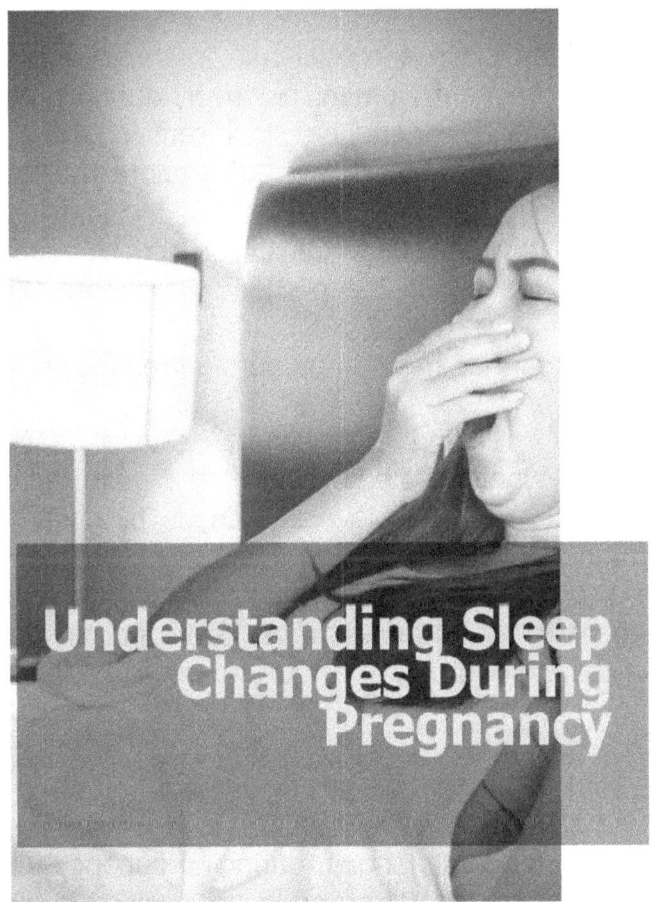

Understanding Sleep
Changes During
Pregnancy

Chapter 1: Understanding Sleep Changes During Pregnancy

Sleep plays a crucial role in the health and well-being of pregnant women, however, during pregnancy, it is common to experience significant changes in sleep patterns. In this chapter, we will explore the factors that affect sleep during pregnancy, including hormonal changes, physical adaptations, and the emotional effects related to inadequate sleep.

1.1. Factors that affect sleep during pregnancy

During pregnancy, several factors can influence women's sleep. One of the main factors is the increase in hormone levels, such as progesterone. This hormone plays a key role in maintaining pregnancy, but it can also cause excessive drowsiness and dysregulation of sleep patterns. In addition, estrogen and prolactin levels also change, which can affect the quality and duration of sleep.

1.2. Hormonal changes and their impact on sleep

Hormonal changes during pregnancy can affect sleep patterns in different ways. Excessive drowsiness may occur, especially during the first trimester, due to increased levels of progesterone. On the other hand, hormonal changes can lead to difficulties falling asleep and staying asleep, resulting in fragmentation and insomnia.

1.3. Physical adaptations and discomforts that can interfere with sleep

As pregnancy progresses, significant physical adaptations occur in a woman's body. The enlarged uterus can cause discomfort in the back, abdomen and joints, making it difficult to find a comfortable sleeping position. Furthermore, increased pressure from the uterus on the bladder can result in increased urination during the night, interrupting sleep.

1.4. Emotional and Psychological Effects of Inadequate Sleep During Pregnancy

Pregnancy is a period full of emotions and worries, which can affect pregnant women's sleep. Concerns about the baby's health, adjustments in family life, anxiety about childbirth and changes in life after birth can lead to difficulties falling or staying asleep. Nighttime stress and anxiety can contribute to an unsatisfactory sleep cycle and negatively affect pregnant women's mental health.

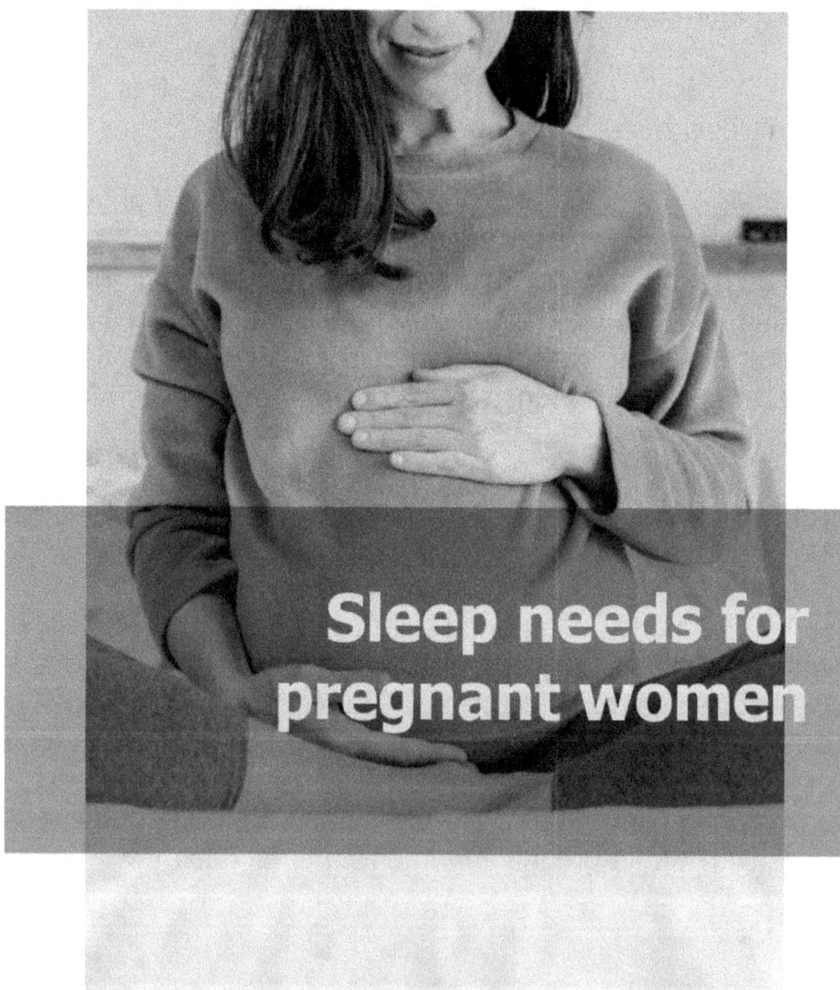
Sleep needs for
pregnant women

Chapter 2: Sleep needs for pregnant women

2.1. Optimal Sleep Duration During Pregnancy

During pregnancy, sleep needs may vary from woman to woman and throughout the different stages of pregnancy. However, experts recommend that pregnant women aim to sleep 7 to 9 hours a night. This adequate sleep range is essential for providing the body with adequate rest and recovery, as well as promoting healthy cognitive and emotional functioning.

2.2. Sleep quality and its benefits for maternal and fetal health

Sleep quality plays a crucial role in the health and well-being of pregnant women and fetal development. During sleep, the body carries out repair and regeneration processes, which is particularly important during pregnancy when significant physical and hormonal changes occur. Good quality sleep is associated with benefits such as:

Strengthening the immune system: adequate sleep supports immune function, helping to prevent infections and illnesses during pregnancy.

Hormonal regulation: quality sleep contributes to adequate hormonal balance, essential for the healthy development of pregnancy and maternal well-being.

Mental and emotional health: Adequate sleep plays a crucial role in the mental health of pregnant women, helping to reduce the risk of depression, anxiety and other emotional disorders.

Cognitive function: Good sleep quality is associated with better cognitive functioning, including memory, concentration and executive performance, which is essential during pregnancy when the expectant mother needs to deal with several important tasks and decisions.

2.3. Sleep patterns and circadian rhythm in pregnancy

During pregnancy, changes may occur in pregnant women's sleep patterns and circadian rhythm. It is common to experience excessive sleepiness during the day, especially in the first trimester, due to hormonal changes. Additionally, sleep fragmentation can occur due to increased urinary frequency and physical discomfort. Understanding these changes in sleep patterns is important to adjust your routine and adopt strategies that promote more restful sleep.

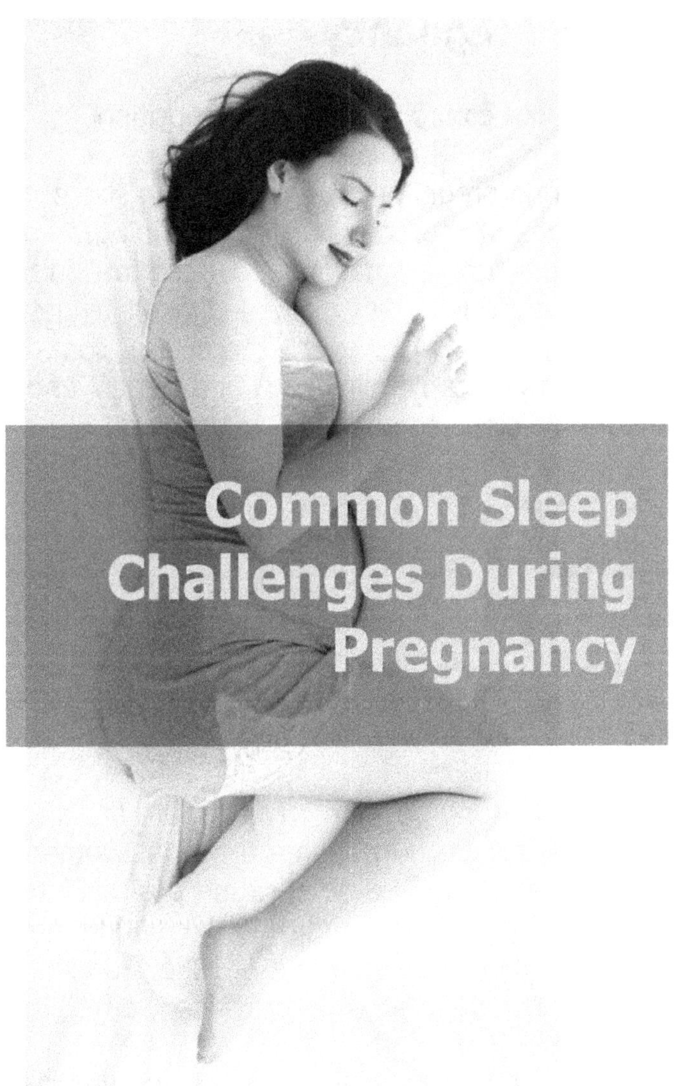

Common Sleep
Challenges During
Pregnancy

Chapter 3: Common Sleep Challenges During Pregnancy

3.1. Finding a comfortable sleeping position

During pregnancy, the increase in size of the uterus and changes in the body can make finding a comfortable sleeping position a challenge. Discomfort in the back, abdomen and joints can make it difficult to get a restful, revitalizing sleep. However, there are some tips and positions that can help you find relief and a more comfortable sleeping position:

Sleeping on your side: The recommended position for pregnant women is to sleep on your side, preferably on the left side. This position helps improve blood flow to the uterus and baby, as well as facilitating kidney function and preventing compression of the inferior vena cava. Place a pillow between your legs to align your spine and relieve pressure on your hips and back.

Semi-sitting position : To alleviate the discomfort of acid reflux or heartburn, some pregnant women may find comfort in sleeping in a semi-sitting position . Use pillows to support your back and head, creating an elevated angle. This helps prevent the backflow of stomach acid into the esophagus and provides some relief from discomfort .

Use supportive pillows: Using strategically placed pillows can help you find a more comfortable sleeping position. Place a pillow between your legs to align your spine and reduce discomfort in your hips and back. You can also place a pillow under your abdomen to provide additional support. Experiment with different settings and adjustments to find the position that works best for you.

Avoid sleeping on your back: In the third trimester, avoid sleeping on your back, as this can cause pressure on the inferior vena cava, impairing blood flow to the uterus and baby. If you wake up on your back, turn to your left side again.

Try a full-body pillow: Full-body pillows designed specifically for pregnant women can provide extra support and comfort while sleeping. These pillows are designed to hug your body, providing support for your abdomen, back, and legs. They help relieve pressure on joints and can be adjusted to suit your individual preferences.

Remember that every woman is unique, and it may take time to find the most comfortable sleeping position during pregnancy. Experiment with different positions and adjustments until you find what works best for you. If you have any concerns or significant discomfort, consult your doctor or midwife
for personalized guidance on the best sleeping position based on your individual condition.

Adequate and comfortable sleep is critical to your well-being during pregnancy. By finding a comfortable sleeping position, you will be able to rest properly and enjoy a more restful and revitalizing sleep routine, thus promoting a healthy and satisfying pregnancy.

3.2. Dealing with increased urinary frequency

During pregnancy, it is common to experience an increase in urinary frequency due to hormonal changes and the growth of the uterus, which puts pressure on the bladder. This frequent need to urinate can interrupt sleep and make it difficult to get a restful night. However, there are some tips and strategies that can help deal with increased urinary frequency:

Drink fluids in moderation at night: Reduce your fluid intake a few hours before bed, especially those that can have a diuretic effect, such as teas or coffee. Avoiding excessive fluid consumption before bed can help reduce the need to urinate during the night.

Empty your bladder completely before bed: Make sure you urinate completely before going to bed. This way, you can empty your bladder as quickly as possible. as much as possible and reduce the need to wake up during the night to urinate.

Avoid holding in urine: When you feel the urge to urinate, go to the bathroom immediately. Holding urine can irritate the bladder and increase urinary frequency even more. Respond to your body's needs and go to the bathroom whenever you feel like it, even if it's at night.

Give preference to underwear and loose clothing: Tight underwear and clothing can put additional pressure on the bladder, increasing the feeling of urinary urgency. Choose comfortable underwear and loose clothing that does not put pressure on the abdominal area.

Elevate your legs: During the day, elevating your legs can help reduce fluid buildup in your legs and feet, relieving pressure on your bladder. This may result in less need to urinate during the night. When resting, place your legs in an elevated position, using pillows or cushions to support them.

Stay calm and in control: Dealing with increased urinary frequency can be frustrating, but try to stay calm and in control. Remember, this is temporary and part of the pregnancy experience. Take a deep breath and find relaxation techniques that can help calm your mind and body.

Dealing with increased urinary frequency may require patience and adjustments to your sleep routine, but it's important to remember that this is temporary and part of the pregnancy journey. If urinary frequency becomes excessive, accompanied by pain, a burning sensation, or other unusual symptoms, it is important to contact your doctor as it may be indicative of a urinary tract infection or other underlying problem.

Finding strategies to manage increased urinary frequency can help minimize sleep disruptions and promote a more restful, refreshing sleep routine.

Understanding and adapting to these changes is key to taking care of your health and well-being during pregnancy.

3.3. Alleviating physical discomfort during sleep

During pregnancy, it is common to experience physical discomfort while sleeping due to changes in the body and the growth of the uterus. This discomfort can interfere with the quality of sleep and make it difficult to get a restful night. However, there are some tips and strategies that can help alleviate physical discomfort during sleep:

Use support pillows: Using strategically placed support pillows can help alleviate discomfort in different parts of the body. Place a pillow between your legs to align your spine, reduce pressure on your hips and back, and promote a
more comfortable posture. You can also try placing a pillow under your abdomen to provide additional support.

Invest in a comfortable mattress: A suitable and comfortable mattress is essential during pregnancy to ensure a peaceful sleep. Opt for a quality mattress that provides adequate support for your body and helps relieve pressure on sensitive areas such as your hips, back, and shoulders.

Do gentle exercises and stretches: Doing gentle exercises and stretches throughout the day can help relieve physical discomfort and muscle tension. Consult your doctor or a healthcare professional for specific guidance on safe exercise during pregnancy. Avoid high-impact exercises or movements that place excessive pressure on the abdomen.

Try different sleeping positions: Finding the most comfortable sleeping position can vary from pregnant woman to pregnant woman. In addition to the side sleeping position, you can try different tilt angles, such as using pillows to elevate your head and torso. Find the position that offers the most relief and comfort for you.

Wear comfortable clothes for sleeping: Opt for loose-fitting sleepwear made from breathable materials, such as cotton, to prevent overheating and heat.
discomfort. Clothes that are tight or made from synthetic fabrics can cause skin irritation and increase the feeling of discomfort.

Practice relaxation techniques: Before bed, take time to relax and calm your mind and body. Practice deep breathing techniques, meditation, gentle stretching, or listen to relaxing music. This can help reduce muscle tension and promote a state of relaxation for more restful sleep.

3.4. Managing nighttime anxiety and worries

During pregnancy, it is common to experience anxiety and worries, especially at night. Physical and hormonal changes, along with expectations regarding motherhood and the future, can contribute to mental restlessness and make it difficult to sleep peacefully. However, there are some tips and strategies that can help manage nighttime anxiety and worries:

Establish a relaxation routine before bed: Take time before bed to relax and calm your mind. Develop a relaxation routine that includes calming activities, such as reading an inspirational book, listening to soothing music, taking a warm bath, or practicing deep breathing techniques. These practices can help calm the nervous system and prepare the body for peaceful sleep.

Write in a journal or brainstorm dump ": Before going to bed, write in a journal or do a " brain dump " to put all your worries, fears and intrusive thoughts on paper. This exercise can help free your mind and ease the emotional burden, allowing you to rest more peacefully.

Practice relaxation and meditation techniques: Learning relaxation and meditation techniques can help calm the mind and reduce anxiety. Try techniques like mindfulness , guided visualization, or breathing meditation to direct your attention to the present moment and cultivate a state of mental tranquility.

Seek emotional support: Sharing your worries and anxieties with a trusted loved one, such as your partner, close friend or healthcare professional, can help ease the emotional burden. They can offer emotional support and different perspectives that can help calm the mind.

Practice self-care: Taking care of yourself is key to managing nighttime anxiety and worries. Set aside time during the day to engage in activities that bring you joy and relaxation, such as gentle exercise, listening to music, reading an inspirational book, or enjoying some quiet time. Prioritizing self-care helps
to strengthen your mental and emotional health, promoting more peaceful sleep.

Limit exposure to negative news and media: Excessive exposure to negative or stressful news can increase anxiety and worry. Try limiting your exposure time to these sources before bed and choose more positive, uplifting content.

Learn stress management techniques: Identifying and applying stress management techniques can be helpful in dealing with nighttime anxiety. Try deep breathing exercises, gentle yoga practices, creative activities such as drawing or painting, or even listening to relaxing music. Find what works best for you and incorporate these techniques into your daily routine.

Dealing with nighttime anxiety and worries can take time and practice, but it's critical to prioritize stress management and self-care to promote more restful, restful sleep during pregnancy. If anxiety and worries persist and significantly interfere with your quality of life, consider seeking support from a mental health professional for additional guidance and support.

By implementing these strategies, you will be taking care of your mental and emotional health, creating an environment conducive to more restful, revitalizing sleep , and promoting a healthier, more satisfying pregnancy experience.

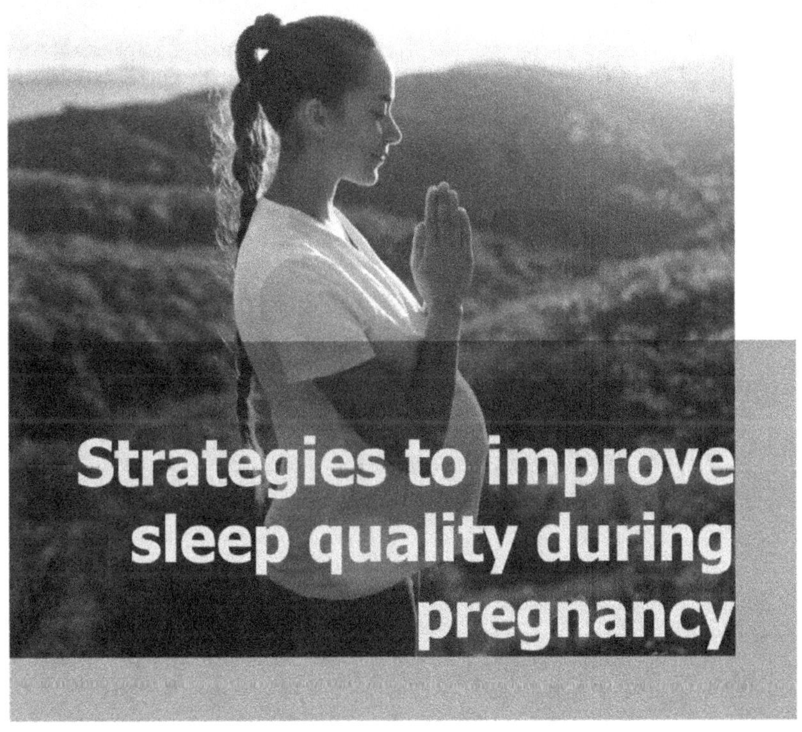
Strategies to improve
sleep quality during
pregnancy

Chapter 4: Strategies to improve sleep quality during pregnancy

4.1. Establishing a Healthy Sleep Routine

A consistent sleep routine is essential for regulating the body's internal clock and promoting healthy sleep. It is recommended to establish regular bedtimes and wake-up times, even on weekends. Maintaining a consistent schedule helps your body prepare for sleep, making it easier to fall asleep and stay asleep throughout the night.

4.2. Creating an environment conducive to sleep

A quiet and comfortable environment can make all the difference in the quality of your sleep. Make sure the room is dark, quiet and at an appropriate temperature. Use curtains or eye masks to block outside light, use ear plugs to minimize unwanted noise, and adjust the room temperature to a pleasant, cool level.

4.3. Relaxation and stress reduction techniques

Practicing relaxation techniques before bed can help calm your mind and body, preparing you for a restful night's sleep. Deep breathing exercises, meditation, gentle yoga, or reading a book
Relaxing are some options that can be incorporated into your nighttime routine. Avoid stimulating activities, such

as the use of electronic devices, in the hours before sleep, as they can interfere with relaxation.

4.4. Exercises and physical activities recommended for pregnant women

Regularly practicing light exercises suitable for pregnant women can contribute to better sleep quality. Consult a healthcare professional for specific guidance on the most appropriate exercises for your condition. Exercises such as walking, swimming, prenatal yoga and gentle stretching can help relax muscles, relieve stress and promote more restful sleep.

4.5. Balanced diet to promote restful sleep

A healthy, balanced diet is important for general health and can also affect sleep quality. Avoid heavy meals before bed as they can cause digestive discomfort. Opt for light, nutritious foods such as fruits, vegetables, whole grains and lean proteins. Also, avoid consuming caffeine and stimulant drinks at night, as they can interfere with sleep.

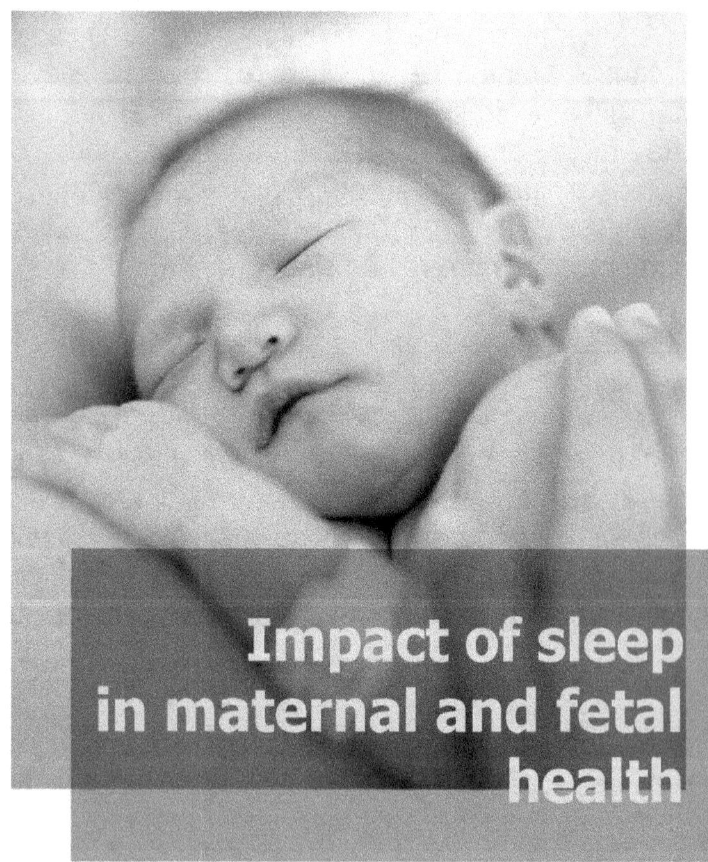
Impact of sleep
in maternal and fetal
health

Chapter 5: Impact of sleep on maternal and fetal health

5.1. Gestational complications related to inadequate sleep

Chronic sleep deprivation during pregnancy has been linked to an increased risk of pregnancy complications. Studies show that a lack of adequate sleep can increase the chances of developing preeclampsia, a condition characterized by high blood pressure and damage to organs such as the liver and kidneys. Additionally, sleep deprivation can also increase your risk of developing gestational diabetes, a glucose metabolism disorder that occurs during pregnancy.

5.2. Mental health and emotional well-being during pregnancy

Sleep quality plays a crucial role in the mental and emotional health of pregnant women. Sleep deprivation can contribute to the development of symptoms of depression, anxiety and stress during pregnancy. Emotional instability resulting from lack of adequate sleep can negatively affect quality of life and relationships with partners and family. It Is essentlal that pregnant women seek support and guidance
appropriate if they are experiencing emotional difficulties related to sleep.

5.3. Fetal development and influence of maternal sleep

Adequate sleep for pregnant women can also have an impact on the development and well-being of the fetus. Studies show that sleep deprivation during pregnancy is associated with a higher risk of low birth weight and premature birth. Furthermore, maternal sleep quality can also influence fetal activity patterns. Inadequate sleep can lead to a reduction in fetal activity, which may indicate problems with the baby's development and well-being.

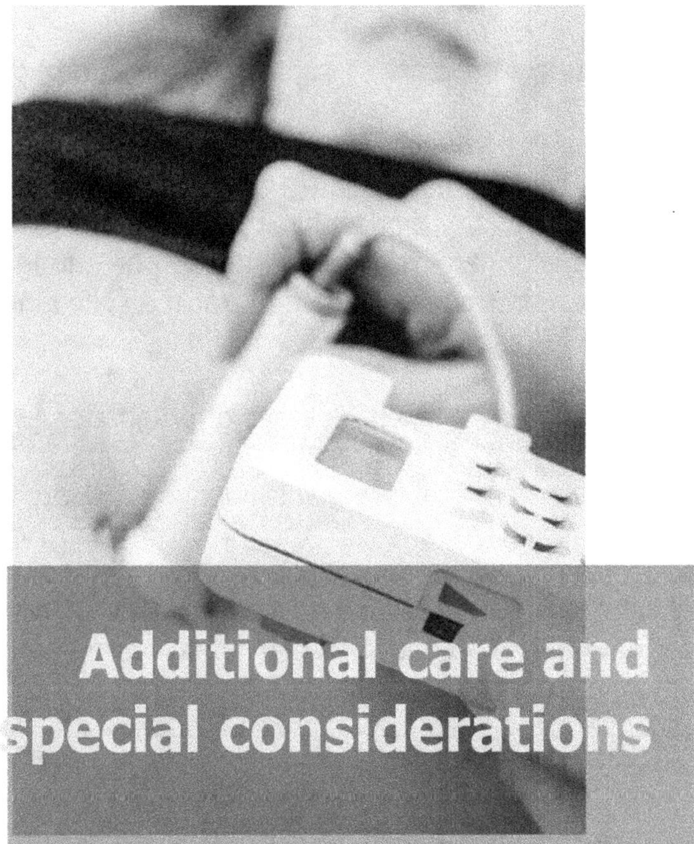
Additional care and
special considerations

Chapter 6: Additional Care and Special Considerations

6.1. Partners and family support in sleep routine

During pregnancy, support from your partner and family plays a fundamental role in pregnant women's sleep routine. A partner can help create a peaceful sleeping environment, share household chores to reduce stress, and offer emotional support. Additionally, having someone to share the responsibilities of caring for the baby after birth can help ensure that the pregnant woman has time to rest adequately.

6.2. Guidelines for specific stages of pregnancy

Each stage of pregnancy brings unique challenges to your sleep routine. In the first trimester, excessive sleepiness is common, and pregnant women may need to adjust their routine to accommodate naps or rest during the day. In the second trimester, many women experience an increase in energy and can take advantage of this by establishing a regular exercise routine. In the third trimester, physical discomfort is more pronounced, and finding a comfortable sleeping position can become more challenging. Understanding these changes and adapting your sleep routine accordingly is essential to ensuring adequate rest.

6.3. Medical consultations and professional support

It is important to seek appropriate medical advice during pregnancy, especially regarding sleep. The obstetrician or midwife can provide personalized guidance based on the pregnant woman's individual needs. If there are significant concerns or difficulties regarding sleep, the healthcare professional can evaluate and offer appropriate treatment options, such as behavioral therapy, suggested adjustments to routine, or, in specific cases, referral to a sleep medicine specialist.

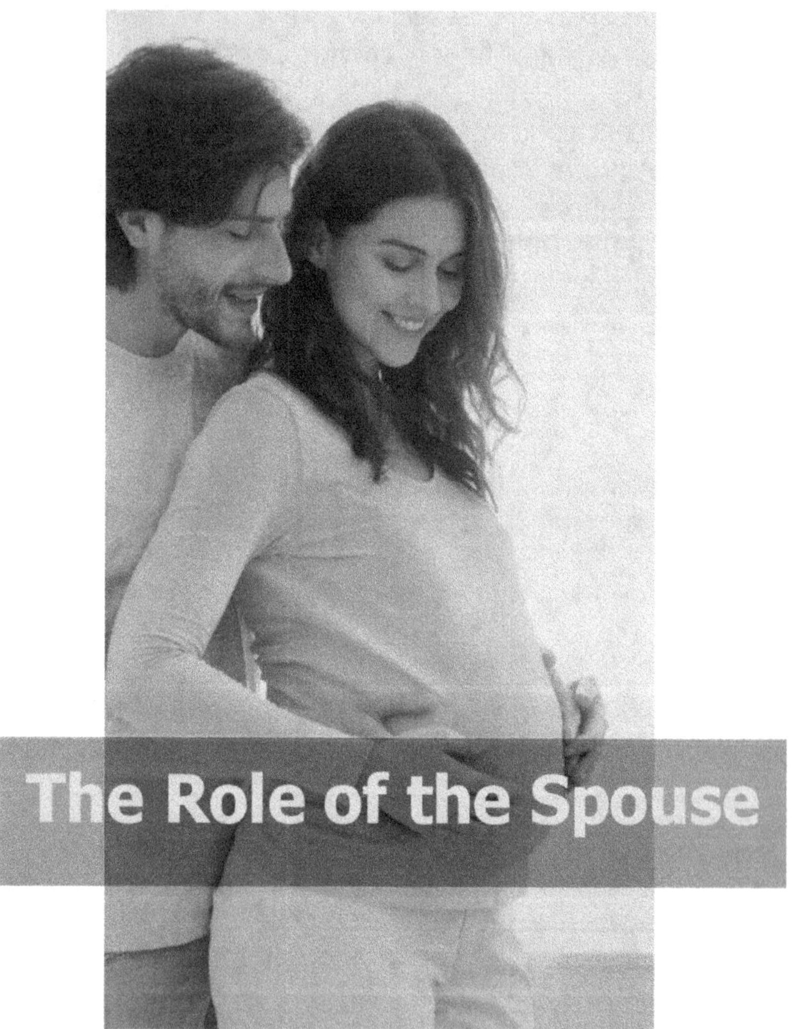
The Role of the Spouse

Chapter 7: The Role of the Spouse: Support in Creating and Maintaining an Optimal Sleep Pattern

7.1. Understanding and patience

The spouse plays a fundamental role in offering understanding and patience to the pregnant woman. Pregnancy brings physical and emotional changes, which can affect sleep and lead to a need for extra rest. By demonstrating understanding and patience, the spouse can help alleviate stress and anxiety, providing a conducive environment for the pregnant woman to sleep peacefully.

7.2. Share responsibilities

A practical and effective way to support pregnant women is to share household and baby care responsibilities. By taking on tasks such as meal preparation, cleaning and laundry, the spouse lightens the pregnant woman's burden, allowing her more time to rest and sleep properly. This division of tasks is a valuable and essential show of support for promoting healthy sleep.

7.3. Offer emotional assistance

Pregnancy can be an emotionally challenging time, and a spouse can play a vital role in providing emotional support to the pregnant woman. Listen to your worries and anxieties, being emotionally supportive and providing words of encouragement are effective ways to help reduce stress and anxiety, which contributes to more restful and restful sleep.

7.4. Participate in creating a sleep routine

A spouse can play an active role in creating a healthy sleep routine for the pregnant woman. This may include establishing a regular bedtime and wake-up time, creating a calm and comfortable environment in the bedroom, and helping the pregnant woman relax before bed through quiet activities such as reading a book or listening to relaxing music. The spouse's participation in this process strengthens support and collaboration in the search for quality sleep.

7.5. Provide a suitable sleep environment

The spouse can play an active role in creating a suitable sleep environment. This includes ensuring the room is dark, quiet and at a comfortable temperature, as well as helping to minimize external noise that may disturb the pregnant woman's sleep. By collaborating in creating an environment conducive to sleep, the spouse contributes to a more peaceful and revitalizing rest.

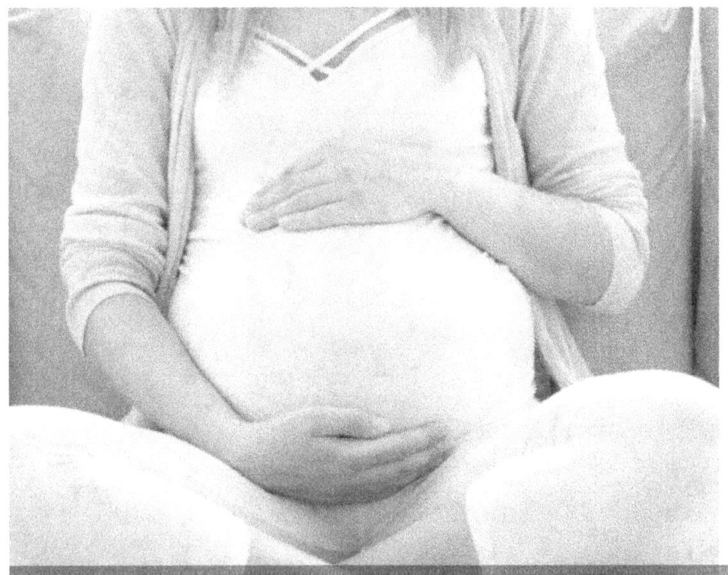
Preparing for the
baby's arrival:
Postpartum sleep

Sleeping for Two, by Ana Maria Santos

Chapter 8: Preparing for the baby's arrival: Postpartum sleep

As you approach the end of your pregnancy, it's important to start preparing for your baby's arrival and understand the changes that will occur to your sleep routine in the postpartum period. In this chapter, we'll discuss realistic expectations about sleep after your baby is born, strategies for coping with sleep deprivation, and the importance of self-care during this time.

8.1. Realistic expectations about postpartum sleep

After your baby is born, your sleep pattern will be significantly altered. Newborns have constant needs for feeding, diaper changes and comfort, which results in frequent awakenings during the night. It's important to understand that sleep deprivation is a normal part of this phase and that fully recovering from sleep may take some time. Maintaining realistic expectations will help you adapt better to this new routine.

8.2. Strategies for coping with sleep deprivation

Although sleep deprivation can be challenging, there are strategies that can help you deal with it. One option is to share the responsibilities of caring for the baby with a partner or other family members, allowing that you have regular sleep breaks. Taking short naps during the day whenever possible can also help compensate for lack of sleep at night. Additionally, establishing a sleep routine for your baby can help create more predictable patterns and make the falling asleep process easier.

8.3. Self-care during the postpartum period

In the postpartum period, it's easy to focus entirely on caring for your baby and neglect self-care. However, taking care of yourself is essential to maintaining your physical, mental and emotional health. Take time to rest and sleep whenever possible, even if it's just short bursts of time. Additionally, seek emotional support and share your experiences and challenges with other mothers or support groups. Practicing relaxation techniques, such as meditation or deep breathing, can help reduce stress and promote relaxation.

8.4. The importance of seeking help when necessary

Dealing with sleep deprivation and the demands of a newborn can be emotionally challenging. It is essential to recognize that it is normal to feel overwhelmed, sad or anxious at times. If these feelings persist or significantly interfere with your health and well-being, do not hesitate to seek professional help. Talk to a doctor,
A nurse, midwife or psychologist can be extremely beneficial in receiving the support you need during this transition phase.

Conclusion

The arrival of your baby is a special and transformative moment in your life. While sleep can be a challenge in the postpartum period, remember that this phase is temporary and that you are doing an amazing job caring for your little one. With patience, support and self-care, you will be able to get through this phase and eventually find a new balance between your baby's needs and your own well-being.

Congratulations on preparing yourself and seeking knowledge to provide the best care possible for you and your baby. We wish you a motherhood filled with moments of joy, love and refreshing rest.

We have reached the end of this book "Sleeping for Two: A Guide to a Healthy Sleep Routine During Pregnancy". Along this journey, we explore common sleep challenges pregnant women face, pregnancy-specific sleep needs, and practical strategies for improving sleep quality.

Throughout the pages, you learned about the factors that affect sleep during pregnancy, including hormonal changes, physical adaptations, and the emotional effects related to inadequate sleep. Understanding these challenges is essential to adopting effective strategies that promote healthy sleep and general well-being during this special phase of your life.

We discuss the importance of establishing a healthy sleep routine, creating an environment conducive to rest, practicing relaxation techniques, adopting adequate exercise and maintaining a balanced diet. These strategies can help improve sleep quality and contribute to your maternal health and your baby's healthy development.

We also cover additional care and special considerations, such as family and partner support in your sleep routine, guidelines for each stage of pregnancy and the importance of seeking appropriate medical advice.

Remember that each pregnancy is unique, and it's important to listen to your body and adapt recommendations to your individual needs. Seeking adequate emotional and professional support is essential throughout this journey.

We hope that the information and strategies shared in this book have been valuable to you. We hope you enjoy a restful and revitalizing sleep routine during pregnancy, promoting your and your baby's well-being.

We congratulate you for investing time and effort in searching for information that contributes to a
healthy pregnancy and a peaceful sleep routine. Enjoy this special time in your life and we wish you and your baby lots of happiness and health. Good nights sleep and a motherhood full of wonderful moments!